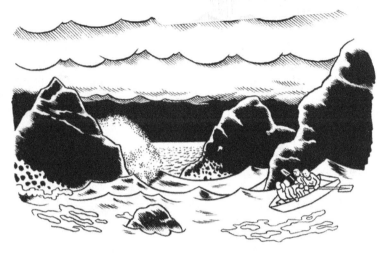

Survive FBT

Skills Manual for Parents Undertaking
Family Based Treatment (FBT)
For Child and Adolescent
Anorexia Nervosa

Maria Ganci

Published in Australia by
LMD Publishing
Melbourne, Australia

First published in Australia 2016
Copyright © Maria Ganci 2016

National Library of Australia Cataloguing-in-Publication entry
Ganci Maria, author
SURVIVE FBT: A Skills Manual for Parents Undertaking Family Based Treatment (FBT) for Child and Adolescent Anorexia Nervosa.
Amanda Spedding, editor
ISBN: 978-0-9944746-9-8 (paperback)
ISBN: 978-0-9944746-2-9 (epub)

Subjects: Eating disorders – Treatment – Anorexia Nervosa – Anorexia in children – Patients – Family relationships. Anorexia in adolescence – Patients – Family Relationships.
Dewey Number: 616.8526

Cover photography by Squishface Studios
Cover design by video_intropro
Illustrations by Ben Hutchings, Squishface Studio
Typesetting by iPublicidades
Printed by Ingram Spark

Disclaimer
All care has been taken in the preparation of the information herein, but no responsibility can be accepted by the publisher or author for any damages resulting from the misinterpretation of this work. All contact details given in this book were current at the time of publication, but are subject to change.

The advice given in this book is based on the experience of the individuals. It is expected that indivduals are engaged in FBT therefore the professionals involved with the family should be consulted for individual problems. The author and publisher shall not be responsible for any person with regard to any loss or damage caused directly or indirectly by the information in this book.

Please do not copy or distribute this material without contacting the author. Last updated July 2015.

ABOUT THE AUTHOR

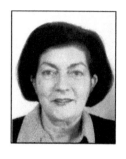 **MARIA GANCI** is a registered Clinical Mental Health Social Worker and Child & Adolescent Psychoanalytic Psychotherapist. Maria's interest in eating disorders commenced in 2005, and in 2007 was one of the founding members of the Specialist Eating Disorders Program at the Royal Children's Hospital, Melbourne. Since that time she has focused solely on providing Family Based Treatment (FBT) and Adolescent Focused Treatment (AFT). Her commitment to families led her to complete a Graduate Certificate in Nutrition at Deakin University.

While working in the Specialist Eating Disorder program, Maria Ganci became the lead FBT therapist in a Randomized Controlled Trial comparing the efficacy of two treatments for adolescent Anorexia Nervosa – Family Based Therapy and Parent Focused Therapy under the guidance of Prof. Daniel LeGrange and Dr Katharine Lobe, both international experts in the field of eating disorders.

In 2014 Maria Ganci was accepted as a faculty member of the Training Institute for Child & Adolescent Eating Disorders, Chicago, USA and currently provides accredited FBT supervision, training and consultation. For further information visit her website www.FBTcentral.com.au.

This book is dedicated to all the families who are enduring the difficult journey towards recovery. I hope this book will give you the knowledge, strength and courage to complete your journey.

ACKNOWLEDGMENTS

Over the years of treating and researching Anorexia Nervosa, many parents have continuously asked me for more information to help them understand anorexia's grip on their child and also to understand how to help their unwell child recover.

This manual was born from those requests and has been written specifically for parents who are undertaking Family Based Treatment for Anorexia Nervosa with their adolescent child. It is based on knowledge gathered from many years of practical experience and research on what makes treatment successful including what parents can do, and must do, to promote their child's recovery.

I sincerely thank the hundreds of families whom I have guided through FBT, without whose experience, this manual would not be possible. It is they who have worked with me and allowed me to learn from them as I have shared their pain and success. I am forever grateful to you all. Particular thanks to the families who have contributed their advice and reflections to this manual.

Just as treating Anorexia Nervosa requires a team approach to support the family, a therapist also requires the support of colleagues and their organization therefore I thank all my colleagues at the Royal Children's Hospital for their continual support. I am also grateful for all the opportunities offered to me by the organization to extend my skills. Sincere thanks to Professor Daniel LeGrange and Dr Katharine Lobe for their tireless and patient supervision which has always led me to reflect and explore my work further. Special thanks to Dr Linsey Atkins, with whom I commenced and continue my FBT journey, for her continual support and inspiration.

A special thanks to my editors Amanda J Spedding and Julie Postance for their endless advice, and without whom this book would not have been possible.

Last but not least, to my wonderful family who have always supported me through all the ventures I have undertaken.

There is always room for improvement, and if parents feel that this manual can be improved by their personal experience to help others, please send me an email at mariaganci84@gmail.com. Also please feel free to visit my website www.fbtcentral.com.au.

FOREWORD

It is hard to imagine a more difficult parenting experience than having to help your child recover from an eating disorder. The combination of medical risk, adolescent resistance, and parental persistence required places you in a unique situation that will test any parent. It must have been all the more difficult in earlier times when professionals emphasized the family as part of the problem rather than the solution. Luckily, it has become increasingly clear over the last 30 years that families are a key resource to help bring about recovery from anorexia, and that this can bring about long-lasting change. This does not take away the experience of feeling the task is overwhelming and stressful, but you can rely on the research evidence behind *Family Based Treatment*, and that other families have gone before you in this endeavor.

Survive FBT is an important resource to help you cope with, and begin treatment with reminders about the key directives that will help you get your child well. You will find in these pages consistent advice to work together as parents, to learn to feed your child the volume and type of food they need, and to help them cope with the experience of treatment. It will also remind you to look after yourself so that you can bring your family back to their normal routines and activities as soon as possible.

Survive FBT provides practical, direct and expert advice that is easily understood and will compliment your therapy appointments. You can trust that the advice in *Survive FBT* is coming from the pen of an experienced therapist who has helped many families through the treatment process.

Mr Andrew Wallis

Co-head, Eating Disorder Service, The Children's Hospital, Westmead, Australia

Faculty Member, Training Institute for Child and Adolescent Eating Disorders

THE JOURNEY

This manual is designed to assist and support parents as they embark on their journey of restoring their child's health. To most parents the journey will feel like sailing through unchartered waters in stormy weather hoping to reach a far-off destination. Most parents commence their journey with minimal sailing skills and feeling very doubtful if they will ever reach their destination.

They are given a map called Family Based Treatment (FBT), which is also foreign to them and outlines what seems to be very strange parenting practices that contradict many of their firmly-held beliefs of parenting which, prior to their child's illness felt logical, comfortable, and served them well.

They are told the journey will be intense and they will need to complete it quickly in order to give their child the best chance of reaching the destination safely and in good health.

The FBT journey is indeed difficult for most parents as their child will not want to travel the journey with them and will desperately try to sabotage their heroic efforts.

Parents will need to put all their faith in the treatment and in their own abilities to get to the destination. The journey is demanding and will require all their energy and internal resources. The greater the commitment to adhering to the FBT map without straying off course, the greater their chance of reaching the destination.

Most parents complete the journey despite all the obstacles and stormy weather along the way. When they reach their destination they are grateful that the healthy child they once knew has returned. Their life can now return to normality. All parents say that this journey was the most difficult thing they have ever done in their life.

Only parents have the determination and courage to complete this journey because it is their love for, and bond with their child that will give them the stamina to succeed.

COURAGE & STRENGTH
ON YOUR JOURNEY

TABLE OF CONTENTS

WHAT IS ANOREXIA?

Anorexia Nervosa is an eating disorder that affects a large number of adolescents, both male and female. Onset is usually around 15-19 years of age for females, and 17-26 years of age for males.* Current figures estimate approximately 1 in 100 adolescent girls will develop anorexia and the ratio of males to females is 1-10.* Anorexia is a mental illness with severe medical complications. This makes it a devastating illness with one of the highest mortality rates of any psychiatric disorder. The mortality rate for Anorexia Nervosa increases for each decade that an individual remains unwell.

Anorexia means "loss of appetite", however this cannot be further from the truth as the loss of appetite is initially self-imposed and mentally driven, and symptoms escalate to the point where the adolescent has minimal ability to return to normalized eating without parental support.

The main features of anorexia are a preoccupation with body image leading to a drive for thinness together with an extreme fear of gaining weight. This is accompanied with a preoccupation of thoughts about food, calories, and weight. For many adolescents symptoms initially commence with a preoccupation with "healthy eating." Whilst their focus on health may initially make sense to their parents, the preoccupation quickly becomes "unhealthy" as they reduce their calories to unsustainable levels that cannot support normal development and daily activities.

In order to maintain a low body weight adolescents will engage in food restriction – either all food groups or selective food groups. Many adolescents also engage in purging behaviors which can be vomiting, laxative use, diuretic use, and exercise. It is the low body weight and these dangerous behaviors that lead to serious medical complications.

Adolescents who have not lost sufficient weight to meet the weight criteria for anorexia but have all the symptoms of anorexia are usually diagnosed as suffering from atypical anorexia. This normally occurs when a large amount of weight has been lost over a brief period of time.

Adolescents who participate in activities and occupations such as dancing, diving, ballet and other activities that require and promote the ideal thin shape seem to have a higher incidence of eating disorders. Anorexia often presents with other psychiatric disorders such as depression, anxiety, and obsessive-compulsive disorder.

We do not know why some adolescents develop Anorexia Nervosa or an eating disorder but we do know that:

AGE – Younger adolescents have a much better recovery rate than older adolescents. [1]

DURATION OF ILLNESS – Early diagnosis and treatment is critical to recovery. Adolescents with a duration of anorexia less than three years have better recovery rates. The longer the adolescent suffers from anorexia the poorer the prognosis. [1]

EARLY WEIGHT GAIN – Early weight gain of approximately 500g per week in the first four weeks of treatment has also been shown to lead to a better outcome. [2]

*Remember – the quicker your child recovers,
the better their prognosis!*

IMPACT OF ANOREXIA
ON MY CHILD'S BODY

Anorexia impacts on every part of your child's body. The medical complications are a direct result of weight loss and malnutrition and can have long term consequences if the body continues to remain in a starved state.

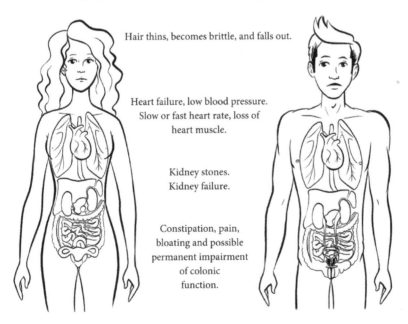

Brain shrinkage, poor concentration and decision making, sad, moody and irritable.

Hair thins, becomes brittle, and falls out.

Heart failure, low blood pressure. Slow or fast heart rate, loss of heart muscle.

Kidney stones. Kidney failure.

Constipation, pain, bloating and possible permanent impairment of colonic function.

Dry skin, bluish discoloration, easy bruisability and delayed wound healing, lanugo (growth of fine body hair).

Cold intolerance as the body has insufficient energy to heat the body.

Peak bone-mass reduction leading to osteopenia and risk of developing osteoporosis long term.

Delayed sexual development or interruption and possible irreversible growth retardation.

Girls – Menstrual dysfunction, loss of periods and possible long term reproduction problems.

Boys – Decreased levels of testosterone, changes in sexual functioning and sexual drive.

Reduced metabolic rate, fatigue, and lack of energy.

Loss of muscle mass, muscle weakness, and swollen joints.

Blood and body fluid problems, anemia, low potassium, magnesium and sodium.

Vomiting can result in dehydration, inflammation and tears of the esophagus, and dental enamel erosion.

IMPACT OF ANOREXIA ON YOUR FAMILY

Apart from the devastating psychological and physiological impact on your child, anorexia can have an overwhelming and distressing impact on the family. The severity of the anorexia and the intensity of the treatment can place many families under enormous stress.

Unfortunately your child's non-compliance will result in many battles between you and your child, and perhaps also battles with your partner if you both do not agree on management strategies.

The continual conflict over food and weight gain may result in your child acting out and their extreme behavior may frighten and distress you given that you have never witnessed your child acting this way.

An important component of the treatment, and a major task for families, is to learn to separate the illness from their child. Parents need to understand that their child is totally driven by anorexic thoughts that will make them non-compliant to the treatment. Accepting this fact will make you realize that it is not your child but the anorexia driving their behavior. It will also help you respond in a more compassionate and blameless manner and less reactive to the non-compliance.

Younger siblings are extremely vulnerable when witnessing high levels of distress, abuse and acting out behavior of their unwell sibling. Some siblings may feel resentful of their unwell sister or brother because they feel their parents have no time for them given that parents must devote the majority of their time to refeeding and attending to their anorexic child.

Despite the demands of FBT on your time it is important to try and maintain the daily routine of siblings so as to minimize any resentful feelings whilst at the same time ensuring that they are included in the treatment. Most siblings worry about the health of their anorexic brother or sister so it is important that they are provided with sufficient information about the illness and treatment and reassured that their ill sibling will be ok.

Some siblings also worry excessively when they see their parents distressed and may worry about the impact on their parents' health. It is important to be aware of these issues, provide reassurance, and speak to your therapist if you have any concerns regarding your anorexic child's siblings.

It also is important that you take care of your own wellbeing. You may need some time out yourself, and ask for support from extended family and friends. Remember the stronger you are mentally, the stronger you will be to fight the anorexia for your child.

WHAT IS FAMILY BASED TREATMENT (FBT)?

Family Based Treatment (FBT) is a manualized treatment for Anorexia Nervosa developed by J Lock & D LeGrange. [1] It is an evidenced-based treatment, which means that it has been tested and shows consistent outcomes of its efficacy. FBT is currently considered to be the best treatment for adolescents under 19 years of age and with a duration of illness of less than three years.

The length of treatment can vary from six to 12 months. Most parents are usually able to restore their child's health during that time. Research shows that there is no difference between a six month and twelve month length of treatment if adhered to correctly. [3]

FBT is divided into three phases of treatment:

Phase 1 – Refeeding and Weight Restoration.

During this time parents are charged with the responsibility of refeeding their child, which means the parents are in control of all food choices, quantity and preparation of meals. Parents will also need to ensure their child does not engage in any exercise and anorexic behaviors that expend energy and calories; therefore constant supervision may be required. These decisions are made with the support and guidance of the FBT therapist. The philosophy underpinning parental control is that the adolescent is unable to manage eating and appropriate food choices because of the strength of the anorexia that dominates and distorts their thinking regarding what is appropriate, healthy nourishment. At this stage of treatment it is erroneous to assume that your child has any insight into his or her illness. The reality is that your child probably believes they are well; is probably reluctant to engage in treatment; and has the desire to remain thin despite your desperate efforts to feed them.

Phase 2 – Returning Control of Eating back to the Adolescent.

As a result of renourishment it is expected that your child's distress and anorexic behaviors will diminish. Hopefully your child will begin to develop some insight into their illness. In Phase 2 your child should be eating a wide variety of foods and feeling more comfortable about eating. Whilst your child's distorted thinking has not completely disappeared (and will take some time to do so), with good weight gain many adolescents are usually able to manage their anorexic thoughts much better. At this stage parents usually report that their child's mood has lifted and they have become more interactive. Many parents feel they are seeing more of their child than the anorexia. These signs of recovery are individual for each child, therefore, commencing Phase 2 may vary with each family. It is during Phase 2, following appropriate signs of recovery, that parents gradually hand back developmentally-appropriate control of eating and choices to their child whilst at the same time helping their child manage lapses in thinking and eating.

Phase 3 – Treatment Completion and Identifying Adolescent Issues that may need to be Addressed.

During this phase it is assumed that the adolescent is weight restored, capable of managing independent eating, and re-engaged in normal adolescent activities. The main focus of this phase is to identify any issues that impede appropriate adolescent development. Your therapist will help you make appropriate plans to address these issues. If your child suffered from pre-existing mental health issues such as anxiety and OCD, these should be treated following FBT. The main goal of this phase is for the family and adolescent to return to a normal life without an eating disorder.

The key features of FBT are:

→ The parents are seen as the agents for change; therefore the treatment aims to empower parents to take charge of restoring their child's health. The assumption is that the parents are the best resource to bring about their child's recovery.

→ FBT takes an agnostic stance. The treatment does not blame anyone for causing the illness nor does the treatment look for any underlying cause for the anorexia. The stance taken in FBT is that your child has anorexia, which is life threatening, so you and your treating team need to get your child better as quickly as possible.

→ FBT externalizes the anorexia. This means the adolescent is not to blame for the anorexia but that the illness has taken over their mind and become so powerful that they are no longer able to rid themselves of the illness, therefore requiring the help of their parents in order to recover.

Your child will have the best chance of recovery if you are able to commit to and maintain the consistency required by the treatment. Diluting or modifying the treatment is not recommended and may negatively impact on the outcome. FBT is a very intense treatment because you will be continually confronted by two major forces.

1. *Your child does not think they are unwell. Their distorted thinking tells them they are just "great" being thin, therefore they have no motivation to change.*

2. *Your child does not want your help and may see you as the enemy who is trying to make them fat.*

FBT IS THE PRESCRIPTION TO GET YOUR CHILD WELL

SICK CHILD – MEDICINE IS PHARMACEUTICALS

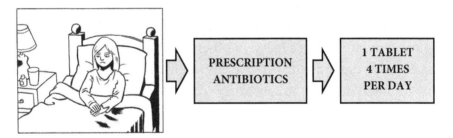

ANOREXIC CHILD – MEDICINE IS FOOD

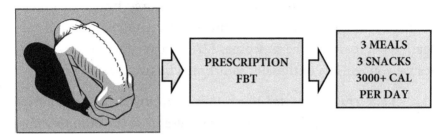

SEPARATING THE ILLNESS FROM THE CHILD

Another core tenant of FBT is separating the illness from your child. Your therapist will help you recognize normal adolescent behavior and behavior that is influenced by the anorexic thoughts. The anorexic behaviors are very foreign, confusing, and distressing for many parents as they are so out of character of their previously healthy child. Once parents are made aware that their child's behavior is driven by anorexic thoughts, it makes it easier for parents to manage the behaviors.

Many adolescents hate parents and/or the therapist making the distinction that it is the illness, not them, driving their behavior and may angrily respond with "It's not the anorexia, it's me" or "This is what I want to do, not the anorexia."

A good and simple analogy to help parents and adolescents understand what the therapist means when they separate the illness from the child is to compare it to your child developing a physical illness/infection. When your child catches a cold she or he is invaded by a virus that makes many changes to their body. Their temperature rises, they may have a runny nose, sore throat, aches and pains etc. They may also lose their appetite, become tired and lethargic, disinterested and unable to concentrate. Whilst it is still your child, they are affected by the virus and will behave very differently under the influence of the virus. Depending on the severity of the virus and viral symptoms they may even become delusional, particularly if their temperature rises too high. This is similar to what happens to your child when they develop anorexia. It is still your child but their behavior is being influenced by the anorexia.

WHAT DOES RECOVERY MEAN?

Full recovery – The Ideal

- ✓ Return to "normalized" eating. This means being able to eat spontaneously and independently when hungry.

- ✓ Ability to eat a wide variety of foods without fear of calories and/or weight gain.

- ✓ Freedom from anorexic thoughts and preoccupations with food and weight.

- ✓ Loving and accepting one's body the way it is despite some "normative discontent" which many people may experience but which does not impact on lifestyle.

- ✓ A return to normal physical growth and development that allows the adolescent to achieve their growth potential. For females this will include a return of menses.

- ✓ Participating in normal adolescent activities such as school, socializing with friends and family, engaging in sport and activities of interest.

Whilst weight restoration may be achieved rapidly, it may take some time for your child to reach full recovery as described above. All adolescents vary in their stage of recovery and much is dependent on their personality traits, length of illness, and pre-existing mental-health issues. For some adolescents, recovery from anorexic thoughts may take 12-18 months. Remember that anorexia is a trauma to the brain, therefore the brain requires time to heal. If your child sustained a complicated and severe leg fracture you would expect that it would take a long time for your child to return to competitive running – the brain probably takes longer given its complexity.

YOUR TREATING TEAM

In order to restore your child's health you will need a team of experienced professionals supporting you through your task of refeeding your child to health. The treatment team consists of the parents, the FBT therapist, the pediatrician, and the psychiatrist.

ROLE OF THE PARENTS – the term "parents" is used but refers to any person who has the responsibility of caring for the child.

Parents are the *most important* team members. They are in charge of their child's recovery and usually know what their child needs given their many years of raising a healthy child. Unfortunately the anorexia has thrown them off their normal parenting path. Parents are the ones who will spend the long hours with their child providing support, understanding, encouragement, love and most importantly – nourishment. Most parents, upon completing treatment, say that this treatment (FBT) is the hardest thing they have ever done in their lives.

The task will be easier if parents can be calm, consistent, patient, available, and creative in the face of a thankless anorexic adolescent who does not want their parents help and who does not want to recover from anorexia given that they love and feel comfortable in their thin body.

Parents are the experts regarding their child.

ROLE OF THE FBT THERAPIST

A therapist's role is to support and guide parents in providing FBT. Your therapist has the expert knowledge about eating disorders and FBT, but cannot **DO** the treatment. Parents are the only ones that can **DO** the treatment.

Your therapist will guide and provide advice regarding the many difficulties you will confront as a parent when refeeding your child and managing many of their anorexic behaviors.

The role of the therapist is also to provide education regarding their child's illness, together with support, encouragement and eliciting belief that their child will recover – given that many parents, upon commencing treatment, may feel that the task ahead is insurmountable. Feeling overwhelmed is a common experience for parents; however, with the support of their therapist, parents usually overcome feelings of hopelessness and get on with their parenting role.

Your therapist will have confidence in you that you can get the job done. Likewise, parents also need to have confidence in their therapist. Parents also need to maintain a strong belief that the treatment will work. Without this mutual confidence and belief, success is usually difficult. Parents are encouraged to question any aspect of treatment they feel they do not understand.

The therapist is the expert regarding FBT.

THE ROLE OF THE PEDIATRICIAN

The role of the pediatrician is to monitor your child's medical status. Given that anorexia is a mental illness with medical complications that can lead to long-term physical damage as well as death, regular medical monitoring is advisable especially in the early stages of treatment when the adolescent has lost a significant amount of weight. The only advice your pediatrician will provide is medical advice. The pediatrician is also responsible for your child's physical development and will request blood tests, bone density tests, or any other tests as required to ensure your child's development remains on track.

> *The pediatrician is the expert regarding medical stability and medical concerns.*

THE ROLE OF THE PSYCHIATRIST

During the early refeeding stage many adolescents experience high levels of distress. Most parents are able to manage this distress with the support of their therapist. However, if your child's distress becomes overwhelming to the point where your child engages in self-harming behaviors or suicidal ideation, a psychiatrist will become involved to review your child, and if required, may prescribe medication. Any decision to prescribe medication for your child will be discussed with you, and you will make the ultimate decision if you wish to place your child on medication. Whilst many of your child's behaviors can be very frightening for parents, they are common in anorexic adolescents and usually subside with weight restoration.

> *The psychiatrist is the expert regarding your child's mental status.*

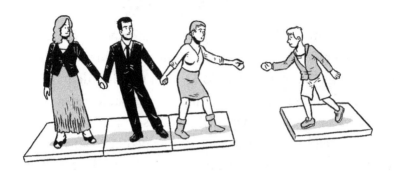

*Remember - the job cannot be completed
without all team members working together!*

REFEEDING MY CHILD

R efeeding an anorexic child is usually the most difficult task for parents undertaking FBT.

Feeding an anorexic child is not normal feeding. Most parents have been very proficient at feeding their healthy child. A healthy child normally has an appetite, normally loves food, and all the brain pathways connected to food and appetite are working efficiently. However an anorexic child does not have an appetite, hates and is fearful of food, and with a starved brain all "food" pathways are disconnected. A healthy child requires sufficient food to provide for growth, metabolic rate and calories expended for exercise. In contrast an anorexic child, whilst requiring similar calories, also requires additional calories for significant weight gain.

Many FBT therapists will usually tell parents that they have the expertise to feed their child and to draw from past experience of feeding a healthy child. Whilst this is usually the case, feeding an unwell and underweight child poses new difficulties for parents. When their child was well and they were presented with a nutritious meal it was quickly and happily devoured. Now anorexia has catapulted them into unfamiliar and terrifying territory. They are confronted with complete food refusal and the accompanying distress from eating. Parents suddenly need to calculate calories and/or quantities of food needed for the required weight gain of 500g to 1kg per week. Many are surprised at the huge quantities required to achieve that weight gain and usually spend many hours planning meals and snacks. Consequently parents usually lose their confidence and begin to doubt their own capabilities and can benefit from assistance managing the dietary requirements for a growing adolescent who is expected to achieve weight restoration quickly.

Knowledge about the impact of under-nutrition on the adolescent body is also foreign to them as they had previously left growth and development to its natural course. Your FBT therapist will guide you in an effort to empower you to get the task done quickly instead of being left to the pitfalls of trial and error.

WHAT MAKES IT SO HARD FOR MY CHILD TO EAT?

Parents struggle to understand why it is so difficult for their child to eat. After all, eating is such a natural instinct and such a pleasurable experience. When parents develop a good understanding of why it is so difficult for their child to eat they are usually able to respond in a much calmer and compassionate manner. They become less frustrated and more patient, and they become more determined to get their child better as quickly as possible to free them from the tormenting distress their child experiences.

The following six factors are what your child is experiencing every minute of every day whilst suffering with anorexia, and it is these factors that interfere with eating and weight gain.

1. Your Child is Scared

The most common underlying emotion of anorexia is FEAR. Your child has what may appear to you an irrational fear of food and eating, but what your child has, is an irrational fear of getting fat. Your child is scared that any food they eat will immediately deposit huge quantities of fat on their body.

Your child is also scared of calories; they are scared of scales, being weighed, and consequent weight gain. They are scared of what their friends will think of them if they gain weight; they are scared that if they start eating "fear" foods they won't be able to stop. They are scared of losing control as anorexia makes them feel in control; they are scared of losing their identity as anorexia has given them an identity, and the list goes on and on.

The fear is so great that it consumes your child's thinking throughout most of the day. Your child continually counts calories, thinks about the horror of the next meal; how they can avoid it; and how they can expend the calories you are giving them. Imagine how hard it must be for your child to eat with all this fear!

2. Your Child is Anxious

Food and the thought of gaining weight makes your child anxious. Current research tells us that many children with anorexia also have a comorbid mood disorder (depression) or anxiety disorder (obsessive compulsive disorder, anxiety disorder or social phobia). Loch (2015) found that 50% of adolescents with anorexia had a mood disorder and 35% an anxiety disorder. [4]

Many parents also report their child was an anxious child pre-anorexia. If your child already had pre-existing anxiety or a mood disorder their symptoms will be exacerbated with anorexia, especially when confronted with food.

Your child's anxiety can become so irrational and extreme that when you put a normal plate of food in front of them they will see a mountain of calories that will immediately be visible on a part of their body they hate. As the anxiety increases so does the rigidity and desperate attempts to control their environment and intake in an effort to reduce the anxiety. Your child will unconsciously think "If I can control the food, I can control my anxiety." For some children their high levels of anxiety can lead to a panic attack.

3. Your Child is Dealing with the Constant Internal Dialogue of Anorexia

Your child is tormented by a barrage of internal dialogue from anorexia. It's a constant voice/thoughts in their head telling them not to eat, and if they eat they will get fat; they will be ugly; nobody will like them if they are fat. The anorexia also tells them not to trust you and that you are against them and only want to make them fat. Anorexia tells them it is their friend and the only friend that can be trusted, the only friend that is faithful to them and has their interests at heart. The anorexia persuades them that it is so faithful to them that *it is* them and becomes their identity. Anorexia also tells your child that life cannot go on without the control and safety it bestows on them, and by eating they will lose that control. Anorexia makes your child believe that they are only special if they remain thin.

Some adolescents do have another small voice telling them they are hurting and upsetting you, and that you really love them and want them to get better, but that voice is so small that it gets drowned out in the background noise of anorexia. Some adolescents say they are trapped in a no-win situation – if they eat to make you happy, the anorexia will chastise/punish them, and if they make the anorexia happy by not eating, you will chastise and get angry with them.

4. Your Child is Governed by Countless Self-imposed Rules

In order to feel safe and in control, your child has developed countless rules that will ensure they don't stray from their goal to remain thin and/or lose weight. These rules make little sense to parents, but to your child they are comforting because if there are rules then there are boundaries to stay within. Rules provide a sense of safety and containment, as do rules in society. The more weight that is lost, the more unwell your child becomes and the more rigid the rules become.

The rules are very similar to the thoughts, but unlike the voices and thoughts that come and go, rules are fixed and must be obeyed at any expense.

→ I must check calories in everything I eat to make sure I won't gain weight.

→ I can only eat _____ calories in a day.

→ I cannot eat fats or carbohydrates.

→ I must exercise/purge to ensure I stay the same or lose extra calories I have eaten.

→ Being a low weight is more important than anything else in my life.

→ I can't eat anything after 7.00 pm.

→ Only by being thin will I be attractive to others.

→ Only by being thin will I be perfect.

→ Only thin people are in control, fat people have no control.

5. Your Child has a Starved Brain

The brain is the most important organ in the body, and therefore the body makes every effort to preserve the brain. During starvation the brain receives priority at gaining access to nutrition at the expense of other organs and body functions. The brain's only fuel source is glucose. When glucose levels are low the body will initially metabolize fat followed by muscle tissue (proteins) in an effort to access glucose. When starvation is severe and prolonged the body will break down neurons to access glucose for the brain, which results in loss of neurons and brain shrinkage.

Brain imaging studies in anorexic patients have shown anatomical features of brain shrinkage, loss of neuronal cell bodies and a reduction in the density of the synaptic connections. The loss of brain matter appears to be reversible with weight gain in most cases, but not all.[6] Longer term effects on learning, behavior, and mood is not well understood and requires further research.

A starving brain functions very differently to a well-fed brain and many of the clinical symptoms seen in anorexia are caused by changes in brain structure secondary to starvation.[5] Starvation leads to an impairment in the frontal lobes responsible for executive functioning – judgment, insight, concentration, and decision making,[6] hence why your child will appear so unreasonable and irrational to you.

The Insula is an area of the brain that appears to become very dysregulated by starvation. The Insula's predominant role is to balance parts of the brain that deal with adaptation to the external environment and those responsible for internal homeostasis/ stability. The Insula also regulates appetite and eating. In anorexia, impairment of the Insula leads to abnormalities in the regulation of appetite and eating, an exaggerated sense of fullness, distortion of body image, difficulties in the integration of thoughts and feelings, anosognosia (unawareness of being ill) and a heightened sense of disgust.[6][7]

6. Your Child may have Certain Personality Traits that Contribute to and Maintain the Illness

Current literature identifies that many adolescents suffering from anorexia appear to share many similar personality traits that appear to either exacerbate or maintain their anorexic symptoms of rigidity and control.

The main traits appear to be:

Perfectionism – Many adolescents set very high standards for themselves. Whatever they do is never good enough – it needs to be perfect; in fact it needs to be flawless. Flawlessness is unachievable, however many adolescents will spend agonizing hours trying to achieve the impossible. Hence their desire to achieve the impossible weight target/body image, which will never be perfect enough for them. Perfectionistic tendencies increase their distress and contribute to the maintenance of the illness.[5]

Cognitive Inflexibility – Cognitive flexibility is the ability to shift between mental sets either cognitively or behaviorally, also known as "set-shifting." Set-shifting is the ability to move flexibly back and forth from one task to another. Difficulties in set-shifting equates to cognitive inflexibility and manifests in concrete and rigid responses that may be linked to behaviors such as compulsive traits, rigidity and perfectionism. Many patients with anorexia seem to have poor set-shifting abilities and get stuck on many maladaptive behaviors even in the face of external pressures being present.[5]

Poor Central Coherence – Central coherence is the ability to see the "big picture." Research on the neuropsychological profile of patients with anorexia has found that they tend to have a detailed, focused processing style often called weak central coherence. This means they tend to focus on detail rather than the bigger picture (detail vs global thinking styles). Lask suggests that this processing style may help us understand the body-image disturbance in anorexics. He hypothesizes that people who get caught up in details in general would also apply this processing style when seeing their own body, hence when a person with anorexia looks at themselves in the mirror they tend to see specific body parts they are unhappy with and evaluate them negatively instead of looking at and evaluating their body as a whole.[5]

ANOREXIC BRAIN

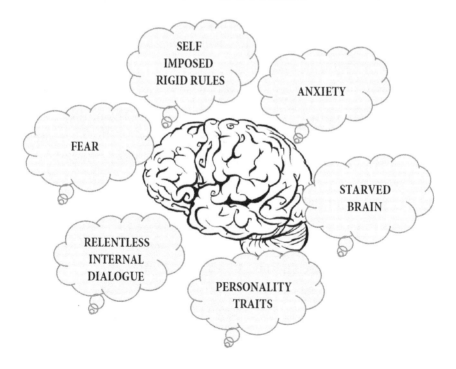

The above factors detail the challenges when feeding your child. It is not a battle with your child, but a battle against fear, anxiety, and ineffectiveness of a starved brain, relentless internal dialogue, and copious self-imposed rules that have possessed your child. Your child **does not** have the resources to undertake this battle on their own; they are powerless against such strong forces. They need **YOU** to battle for them and restore their health, for without you, they will surely be defeated either through death or become a lifelong servant to Anorexia Nervosa. The longer the illness remains, the stronger their identity with anorexia becomes.

FOOD IS MEDICINE

Food is the only thing that will bring about your child's recovery. There are currently no medications that will help your child get better.

Your child's body composition is made up of lean body mass and body fat. Lean body mass refers to the weight of the bones, internal organs, muscles and connective tissues. Body fat refers to essential fat and adipose fat.

Your child's body needs a balance of different nutrients to restore their health. Carbohydrates, proteins, fat, vitamins and minerals are all essential nutrients for your child's body.

Carbohydrates are needed for the body to provide glucose for energy. Glucose is the body's preferred fuel source. Without a good supply of glucose the body will not function effectively. The brain will ONLY use glucose and consumes approximately 30% of the body's required glucose to function. Foods that are high in carbohydrate include breads, cereals, rice, potato, pasta, milk, yoghurt and fruit. Sweets and soft drinks are also high in carbohydrate.

Protein is the body's building material. Protein is not normally used for energy and is only converted when the body does not ingest sufficient carbohydrates. This is an inefficient way to obtain glucose as the body needs to break down protein in order to obtain a small amount of glucose contained in the protein. In anorexia this is called self-cannibalization – the body eats itself to provide glucose to the brain, hence the significant weight loss and muscle tissue wasting. Foods that are high in protein include meat, fish, chicken, milk, yoghurt, cheese, beans, nuts, and seeds.

Fat – Much of the current media hype is that "fats are bad", however the body requires fat to function effectively. Fat should make up 20-30% of total calories. Fat is essential for normal body function. Fat helps the absorption of essential vitamins including vitamin A, D, E and K. Foods that are high in fat include butter and margarine, oils, nuts and seeds, avocado as well as processed foods like take-away and biscuits and cakes.

Fat present in bone marrow, central nervous system, brain, major organs, intestines, and muscles is called essential fat as it is important for normal bodily functioning, as opposed to adipose fat that is accumulated fat when too much fat is consumed. Death from starvation is due to a total depletion of body fat which is used as a reserve for making glucose.

Fat is an essential requirement for a healthy body, and the percentage of body fat in adolescents should be 15-20% dependent on their age and stage of development. Very low body fat can contribute to severe medical complications that involve almost every body function and includes the cardiovascular, endocrine, reproductive, skeletal, immune, gastrointestinal, renal and central nervous systems.

Fat is required for:

→ An insulator to conserve body heat. Low body fat will lead to cold intolerance and low body temperature, hence the reason why adolescents with anorexia are constantly cold.

→ The brain and central nervous system has a high fat percentage. Fat is required as a myelin sheath in the nervous system. Low body fat depletes and destroys the myelin sheath resulting in slow conduction of electrical impulses used by the brain. This results in poor brain functioning, low concentration levels, confusion and irrational thinking.

→ Very low levels of body fat can lead to loss of bone density, which increases the risk of stress fractures.

QUANTITY OF FOOD REQUIRED

Your adolescent will need to eat three meals and three snacks per day totaling to 3000+ calories if they are to gain weight quickly. Some adolescents may need to eat more in the early stages of refeeding because their basal metabolic rate will usually increase. Basal metabolic rate is the rate at which the body uses energy while at rest to maintain vital bodily functions. When people do not eat sufficient calories for some time there is a reduction in their basal metabolic rate and this rate can increase to 120% upon refeeding.

Carbohydrates and fats will usually be your child's "fear" foods as they erroneously believe that if they eat these foods they will get fat. Most adolescents have what they call "safe" foods, however safe foods are usually very low in calories. Your adolescent will not fully recover until they are able to eat all food groups without fear. Consequently, it is your task to ensure your adolescent is presented with both safe and fear foods and consumes a balanced meal containing carbohydrates, proteins and fat.

Many parents fall into the trap of trying to present gourmet dishes and foods in a belief that making food more interesting will entice their child to eat. A child suffering from anorexia will hate most foods so your well-intentioned efforts may not be appreciated. Remember you are not running a restaurant but restoring your child's health. The only thing that is important is to get the right quantity of food into your child to gain weight. Therefore good, wholesome, and nutritious foods should be your main goal. Many parents find that it is easier to increase the calorie density of food (ie. more calories) instead of the quantity, but it will be up to you to find a way to ensure your child has the required calories **every meal, every day** until their physical health is restored.

Following meals your adolescent will complain of feeling full, sick, bloated and having a sore tummy. This is quite normal. During starvation the stomach shrinks a little, and now with the increased intake the stomach will need to stretch and return to its normal size. This discomfort will not last long and a heat bag on their stomach after meals may help.

Many adolescents complain of constipation. This is also quite common and will resolve with normal eating as the digestive system returns to its normal functioning. Whilst water and juice can assist with regularity, it is important to remember that allowing your child to drink too much water will fill your child up and make it more difficult for them to eat their meals.

The adolescent years are the second most intense phase of growth beyond the first year of life. All adolescents require adequate calcium given that adolescence is the time when they accumulate their peak bone density. Osteoporosis is a significant risk factor for adolescents with a prolonged eating disorder. During starvation your child may lose bone density or not accrue bone mass so it is important to get enough calcium in the diet to help replenish it. Teenagers require 3-4 serves of dairy every day. A serve of dairy is: 250ml milk, 200gm yoghurt, 50g of hard cheese such as cheddar or 120g of ricotta cheese. There are many other factors that contribute to strong bone health such as sufficient Vitamin D, and return of menses (estrogen) for females and sufficient testosterone in males. This should be discussed with your pediatrician, who will usually order a bone density test for your child.

Having a diverse community of gut bacteria is important to health, and the latest research suggests that the diversity of the gut microbiota in individuals with anorexia may be reduced possibly due to starvation.[8] Although not tested, a probiotic and/or yoghurt may be useful to restore healthy gut microbes.

Your child's anorexia will also engage in many distracting "food" behaviors parents struggle to understand. Many of the behaviors are to avoid food because it is difficult for your child to eat. They are also an attempt to distract you from your task of refeeding. It is best to stop these behaviors as quickly as possible.

Examples of distracting behaviors are:

- Breaks/cuts food into small pieces
- Smearing food on plate
- Eats with a teaspoon
- Holding food in mouth & not swallowing
- Throwing food/hiding food
- Running away from the table

- Extreme language
- Screaming or crying
- Breaking crockery/furniture
- Attempts to harm themselves with fork, knife etc.

Family meals were videotaped in session two of FBT. Researchers examined the strategies that parents were observed using during refeeding. The videos were analyzed and the interactions were classed into the following categories:

→ Direct eating prompts aimed at directly pressuring the adolescent to eat: "You need to eat all your lunch" or "Pick up the toast and eat it."

→ Non-direct and encouraging eating prompts: "Keep going", "Why don't you eat some more?"

→ Physical prompts: pushing the plate toward the adolescent.

→ Restrictive responses that limited further intake: "That's enough for now." "No more toast now."

→ Positive incentives: "If you finish your meal, you can go to the movies tonight."

→ Negative incentive describing a negative consequence: "If you throw your sandwich on the floor, you will need to eat two."

→ Autonomous comments: "Do you want another one?" or "Which one would you like?"

→ Information provision: "This will make your bones strong."

Interestingly the study showed that parents who used direct eating prompts had the greatest success in getting their child to eat.[9]

MODELLING

Modelling is a process of learning whereby children imitate the behavior of their parents without explicit direction, hence the term role-model.

It will be difficult for your child to eat three meals and three snacks if the family does not model appropriate and normal eating behaviors such as eating regular meals, not skipping meals, eating together as a family etc.

Many families struggle to find a time to eat a family meal together despite their best intentions to do so due to work and sporting commitments. If possible it will usually be easier for your child to eat if you are able to set aside regular meal times with all the family members present to provide support. Eating together also gives the underlying message that eating and meal times are important and are a time to be together sharing and engaging in family conversations.

During mealtimes many adolescents will complain that they are eating more than their siblings and/or their parents. Some parents, in an effort to make it easier for their child, will increase their own or the siblings food intake. This is not advisable and it only reinforces the anorexia's desire for control. Gently tell your child that they are the one who is unwell and that once recovered their intake will be reduced to the quantities of their well siblings.

Most adolescents will be highly anxious about what you are going to feed them, hence they will want to be involved in food shopping, planning and cooking the meals. Having your anorexic child with you during these times will usually result in arguments. Your child will want you to buy low calorie or diet foods and during meal preparation your child will also become anxious and try and convince you not to add high calorie ingredients such as oil, butter etc. Therefore it will be easier for you to shop, cook and plan meals without your child present. Gently explain to your child that you know what their body needs and what you need to do to make them better, also as they recover all choices will be returned to them.

Parents who have suffered from an eating disorder or are currently struggling with an eating disorder may find it extremely difficult to manage and supervise their child at mealtimes. Parents have reported that watching their child eat the quantities of food required triggers past memories of their own eating difficulties. They also report feelings of disgust watching their child eat the large amounts of food required for recovery whilst also acknowledging that their child needs to eat. If you are struggling with this difficulty, do not feel reluctant or embarrassed to raise the situation with your FBT therapist who will help you explore ways to manage refeeding.

Given the strong emphasis in the media on health, wellbeing and weight, many families worry about their weight and shape and many families engage in weight control strategies, diets, restrained eating, health foods and exercise etc. It will be easier for you to manage and refeed your anorexic adolescent if engagement in any of these activities is temporarily suspended until your child recovers. Instead focus on 'normalized' eating, which is eating a variety of foods without fear and eating for pleasure and enjoyment.

EATING OUTSIDE THE HOME ENVIRONMENT

EATING AT SCHOOL

Returning to school and eating at school in front of peers will be a major step for your child. Their anxiety and fear of eating is already high, therefore the thought of eating in front of others and worrying about what others will think of them just compounds their anxiety, making it unbearable.

In Phase 1 of FBT it is recommended that meals at school be supervised by parents. This is to ensure your child is consuming everything you give them and it will probably make it easier for your child to eat. Most parents will organize to eat in the car with their child during the lunch hour. Some parents who are unable to supervise lunches at school will either organize a trusted extended family member or a school teacher to supervise their child. It is not advisable to have siblings or peers supervise meals at school.

If you organize a teacher to supervise lunch you will need to let the teacher know what you have provided for lunch either by photo or email. A better option is to deliver your child's lunch directly to the teacher. Teachers do not know how much your child needs to eat, and unless advised will accept that what your child brings is what you have provided. Do not place your child in a situation to be tempted to throw out portions of their meal as the anorexia may tempt them to do so. Remember that whilst teachers will try their best to help you, they do not have the knowledge about anorexia and investment in your child that you have, therefore, they may easily become distracted with other activities and inadvertently create an opportunity for your child to either hide or throw their food away.

Many adolescents will report that it is difficult to eat with peers as their peers eat very little or not at all. Unfortunately this is very prevalent, therefore you will need to explain to your child that despite this situation you are not responsible for their peers and that you need to do the right thing by your child.

EATING OUT

As mentioned previously, many adolescents are anxious about eating out and in front of others. Going out to a restaurant is daunting for your child because they are fearful of the unknown – what is on the menu; ingredients and calories contained in the food etc. One of the best ways to overcome anxiety is by exposure to the situation/object that creates the anxiety. As your child begins to gradually gain weight you will need to help your child overcome this fear. This is probably best done by planned small steps. Decide beforehand with your child where you will go and what you will order. A small initial step is probably going out for a coffee or something small, and preferably something that your child will eat comfortably. Gradually build up to a meal and challenging foods.

Remember the aim is to return to normalized eating!

TIPS THAT MANY PARENTS REPORT USEFUL WHEN REFEEDING THEIR CHILD

→ It is best to include variety and fear foods right from the start of refeeding, otherwise when you do introduce fear foods it will be like starting all over.

→ Don't get caught in the trap that "healthy food" will get your child better. Anorexia is basically fear of food and, in particular, high-density foods. You will know your child has recovered when they can eat everything without fear, and a good sign of recovery is when they can eat everything they ate prior to anorexia.

→ At meal times don't get into the habit of negotiating, convincing, lecturing, or using logic. It is likely to fail and it's a good tactic anorexia uses to waste/avoid refeeding time. Instead, stick to direct prompting (over and over again) to eat the food you provide your child at meal times as this will wear the anorexia down.

→ Don't fall into the trap of giving your child what you think they will eat. This is accommodating your fear. Give them what they need to get healthy.

→ Don't get your child involved in food preparation, planning, calorie counting with them, shopping or any decisions involving food as their current focus will be on the reduction of calories and eliminating fear foods. Just put the meal in front of your child and provide support.

→ Ensure you know how much your child needs to eat to gain weight and the foods that will achieve good weight gain. Whilst parents are usually very good at knowing what to feed a healthy child, they need to learn quickly how much to feed a starving child.

→ Don't expect that your child will be able to make decisions about what to eat, their thinking is too compromised to do this and they will feel guilty with whichever decision they make. They are in a "no-win" situation and will be relieved when someone makes the decision for them.

→ Try not to talk about healthy eating, but talk about normalized eating. Normalized eating is what the average healthy adolescent does – eats variety, eats regularly, is flexible and eats with enjoyment and without fear.

→ Try and stop all the anorexia behaviors at meal times as quickly as possible, eg. breaking food into small pieces, eating with a teaspoon, etc as these behaviors strengthen the anorexia. Every time you push your child past their fear boundary it will get easier for them (it's like exposure therapy).

→ Be prepared for resistance and a battle with the anorexia. There will be a battle until your child gets the message and believes that you are stronger than the anorexia and that you will not budge because you will not let anything happen to them. The strength of the battle will vary with every family depending on: the strength of the anorexia, your child's personality and characteristics, pre-existing mental health issues such as anxiety and OCD and any family dynamics that arise. The strength of your persistence needs to match the severity of the illness and your child will find your strength reassuring. Learn to be decisive against the anorexia.

→ Don't allow your pet dog to sit with your child whilst eating. Many pets have been fed the meal you thought your child had eaten.

→ Make sure you display parental unity and are both on the same page regarding what your child needs to eat; that the meal is to be completed; that you will not negotiate with anorexia; and that you will back each other up. If anorexia sees any weakness in either parent, it will exploit it.

→ Be vigilant by sitting with and supervising your child to eat the whole meal you provide. You child may hide food up sleeves, in pockets, in serviettes and many places that will surprise you. They will do anything to avoid eating if given half the chance.

→ Despite presenting difficulties, try and make meal times as normal as possible by engaging in family conversations and use distractions.

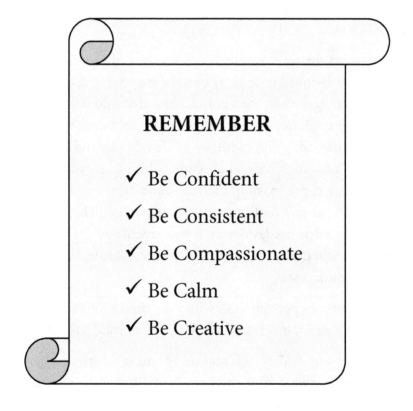

REMEMBER

✓ Be Confident

✓ Be Consistent

✓ Be Compassionate

✓ Be Calm

✓ Be Creative

MEAL AND SNACK PLAN SAMPLES

The following plans provide an example of the quantity of food your child needs to eat for main meals and also what constitutes high-calorie snacks. The meal and snack plan is ONLY a guide to help you understand intake requirements for weight restoration and should be used as such. Feel free to interchange foods of similar calorie content. Your child may prefer to remain on a meal plan; however, it is not a good idea to stick rigorously to the same meal plan every day as it only reinforces rigidity. The goal is for your child to return to normalized eating, which means eating whatever is available and/or served by parents without fear. Research suggests that consumption of a varied diet can be related to improved outcomes in anorexia nervosa.[10]

Sample of appropriate snacks to give your child

(Courtesy of Ingrid Hilton, Dietician)

	MORNING TEA	**AFTERNOON TEA**	**SUPPER**
MONDAY	2 x Anzac biscuits + Apple 250 ml full cream milk or soy milk	1 cup fruit 200g yoghurt, ½ cup toasted granola	350ml milk with 2 tbs Milo + piece of fruit
TUESDAY	'Go Natural' muesli bar 250 ml full cream milk or soy milk	Slice grain toast with tsp butter and banana sliced on top 1 cup milk	300ml milk with 2 tbs milo +2 Anzac biscuits

	Morning Tea	Afternoon Tea	Supper
Wednesday	'Carmens' muesli bar + piece of fruit 250 ml full cream milk or soy milk	Fruit Smoothie (1 banana, 300ml milk, 150g yoghurt full cream, 1 tsp honey, 2 heaped tablespoons oatbran, 2 dates)	Chai powder sachet with 350ml milk tsp honey + fruit
Thursday	Sesame snap bar (40g) + piece of fruit 250 ml full cream milk or soy milk	2 x soy and linseed Vita Wheat lunch slice 2 x 21g cheese + avocado	'Sustagen' tetra pack + piece of fruit
Friday	Cheese/herb scone with tsp butter 250ml milk	1 x Bounce ball + piece of fruit 250 ml full cream milk or soy milk	Hot chocolate 350ml with biscuit
Saturday	1 x fruit/nut bread + butter 250 ml full cream milk or soy milk	1 x 'Emma/Toms' juice 4 Vita Wheat biscuits with 2 tbs nut spread	'Sustagen' tetra pack + piece of fruit
Sunday	1 x dark chocolate and berry muffin 250 ml full cream milk or soy milk	Fruit smoothie (1 banana, 300ml milk, 150g yoghurt full cream, 1 tsp honey, 2 heaped tablespoons oatbran, 2 dates)	350ml milk + 2 tbs Milo + piece of fruit

SAMPLE OF A MEAL PLAN
(Courtesy of Ingrid Hilton, Dietician)

	BREAKFAST	LUNCH	DINNER	DESSERT
DAY ONE	Bowl porridge made with full cream milk/soy (250ml) 1 banana 100g yoghurt 2 tbs LSA 1 tsp honey or brown sugar	Chicken/avoca-do/cheese sandwich (grain bread) 1 glass of juice	Spinach and ricotta cannelloni with parmesan cheese Slice of ciabatta with butter Salad Orange juice	2 scoops ice cream
DAY TWO	2 x slices grain bread 2 x tsp butter 1 tsp vegemite + 1 tsp jam or honey piece of fruit yoghurt	Vegetarian frittata (potato, egg, cheese, milk etc) Salad Glass of juice	Chicken and vegetable stir fry with cashews (oyster sauce or teriyaki) With steamed rice Glass of juice	1 cup yoghurt full cream flavoured + fruit
DAY THREE	1 x Bircher muesli (soaked in 1 x glass fruit juice & yoghurt) 250ml milk 1 banana or mango 1 tsp honey + slivered almonds	Chicken pesto pasta salad with fetta 1 x milk 1x piece of fruit	Lamb/mushroom casserole with mashed sweet potato (made with milk/butter) Steamed vegetables Wholemeal dinner roll with butter Glass of juice	Freddo frog + Glass of milk

	BREAKFAST	LUNCH	DINNER	DESSERT
DAY FOUR	2 x wholegrain toast 2 x butter 2 x eggs ½ avocado 1 glass of milk	Cheese, ham, avocado and tomato toasted sandwich (with butter) 1 x juice	Pan fried salmon or fish Potato/sweet potato wedges Salad with dressing Slice of bread with butter Glass of juice	1 cup full cream custard + piece of fruit
DAY FIVE	2 x Special K (high fiber) 1 banana 250ml full cream or soy milk	Smoked salmon, avocado, cream cheese and salad sandwich Yoghurt Piece of fruit	Roasted vegetable and fetta quiche with salad (dressing) 1 dinner roll with butter Glass of juice	1 cup CALCIYUM
DAY SIX	2 x wholegrain bread 2 x butter 1 x nut butter 1 x jam or honey piece of fruit yoghurt	3 x sushi rolls with avocado/salmon glass of milk piece of fruit	Pasta Bolognaise with parmesan cheese + side salad 1 slice garlic bread Glass of juice	2 scoops ice cream
DAY SEVEN	2 x Weetbix (wholegrain) Banana 250ml full cream milk or soy	Cheese, egg and vegetable quiche with salad Glass of juice	Roast Chicken with gravy Roast potatoes, pumpkin, steamed beans and peas Glass of juice	Slice cheese cake

	BREAKFAST	LUNCH	DINNER	DESSERT
DAY EIGHT	2 x wholemeal toast 2 x butter 1 small tin baked beans Glass orange juice or large piece of fruit	Chicken, egg, cashew nuts and rice salad 1 yoghurt 1 cup of juice	Beef Rendang (coconut curry) with rice or rice noodles 3 papadaams + yoghurt sauce Glass of juice	Cup yoghurt full cream with ¼ cup almonds

Reflections from a Parent –
The Heartache of Refeeding

Prior to refeeding our daughter during FBT, we were at a loss to know how to get her to eat anything outside of her strict self-imposed eating regime. The list of "acceptable" foods was growing less and less and we were very worried and becoming quite desperate.

Our FBT therapist gave us the tools to tackle this frightening illness head-on. We went home and did just that!

Our daughter's distress during refeeding was significant. Whilst it was challenging, frightening and exhausting for us, it was this and so much greater for her. When each "unacceptable" meal was presented, the "thoughts" in her head would scream and rage, so much so that she reacted as if we were expecting her to jump off a 50-meter cliff face. How would you react? Personally, I would fight to the death to stop my parents, in their "naivety", to send me to my destruction.

Our beautiful, caring, co-operative, sensitive, well-mannered, loving daughter quickly became someone else. Her eyes would glaze over and she would throw her food violently and repeatedly as far as she could. She would scream, cry, punch and hit us, throw food at us, throw household items and furniture, swear at us, punch and scratch herself, run around the house, and escape out the front door along streets and alleyways (with us and her siblings chasing behind!). She would often roll herself up into a tight ball so she couldn't eat or didn't have to interact with us. She would hold food in her mouth for up to half an hour and not swallow. She would keep food at the back of her tongue for later disposal. She was adept at hiding food in front of our eyes; in her sleeves, pockets, socks, shoes etc. She would watch my eyes shift momentarily and took the opportunity to hide food. Her distress was so great that she began experiencing suicidal thoughts. We were watching her 24/7 to make sure she did not harm herself.

For many weeks, mealtimes took between 1 to 4 hours from start to finish.

During each meal I would sit next to my daughter and encourage her to eat. I would ask her to pick up her fork and start eating. I would tell her "I know you can do this", "This is what you need", "You're safe, I'm here to help you get through this meal", "Eating is not negotiable, let's keep going now etc." We would ensure she ate the whole meal no matter how long this took. Meals would take many hours but we saw every bite through to the very end. She eventually realized that we would NEVER back down on our expectations and that we would not allow any meal not to be eaten. Yes, we were exhausted but our determination and repetition paid off and eventually she realized it was less tiring for her to eat than to fight against us. We were a strong force and we were determined to "get our daughter back" and save her life.

As parents, keeping calm and "in control" during refeeding was crucial (even though we felt anything but!). Our daughter was so scared and our response had to be calm and reassuring, no matter how difficult that was. She needed our solid reassurance just to be able to cope.

On reflection, we would describe the refeeding process as "exorcising the devil!" It was terrifying but absolutely essential to set our daughter on a path to recovery from Anorexia Nervosa.

Written by a mother of a child, age 9, with Anorexia

ADDITIONAL BEHAVIORS YOUR CHILD MAY ENGAGE IN THAT IMPEDE WEIGHT GAIN

PURGING BEHAVIORS

Purging behaviors are either self-induced vomiting, laxative and/or diuretic abuse. Given the distress and guilt your child may experience following meals they may engage in purging behaviors. This is their attempt to rid themselves of the calories they have consumed and relieve themselves of the guilt.

Purging behaviors have detrimental long-term health consequences, therefore it is advisable to eliminate these behaviors as quickly as possible. Excessive vomiting can cause damage to the esophageal lining, cause reflux, teeth enamel erosion, gastrointestinal bleeding, and electrolyte imbalance. Laxative abuse can cause electrolyte disturbances, can result in weakened pelvic floor and rectal relapse, and interfere with the absorption of nutrients. If your child engages in purging behaviors you will need to monitor them closely, in particular following meals. Bed rest for an hour following meals is usually recommended.] ?

↳ Question for Tammy

48

PHYSICAL ACTIVITY

Many adolescents engage in excessive physical activity in an attempt to expend the calories they have consumed. In the early stage of refeeding it is advisable to suspend all exercise in order to determine how much food your child requires to gain weight. Don't forget your child will be driven to undertake exercise and has very little ability to stop themselves.

Apart from what is normally viewed as exercise there are many forms of exercise your child will engage in that you may not realize is physical activity. Following are examples of activity your child may engage in:

→ Your child prefers to stand than sit – standing consumes more energy than sitting.
   – get your child to sit.

→ Restless hyperactivity – jiggling, walking the long way round to undertake tasks, excessive use of stairs, repetitive unnecessary tasks.
   – stop your child if they engage in these behaviors.

→ Secretive exercise – these occur when your child is unsupervised eg. sit-ups in their room, star jumps/squats in the shower.
   – provide extra supervision and monitoring.

BODY TEMPERATURE   ↘ Discuss w/Tammy

Heating or cooling your body requires energy. Anorexics usually feel cold because of a depleted energy state. Many adolescents with anorexia will try and expend calories/energy by purposefully making themselves either very cold (wearing very light clothing, leaving windows open in cold weather etc.) or making themselves excessively hot to induce sweating (heat their room and cover themselves with a doona – sauna conditions). If you suspect any of these behaviors you will need to ensure your child maintains a normal body temperature to help conserve energy.

Remember you need to be
one step ahead of anorexia!

PARENTAL UNITY

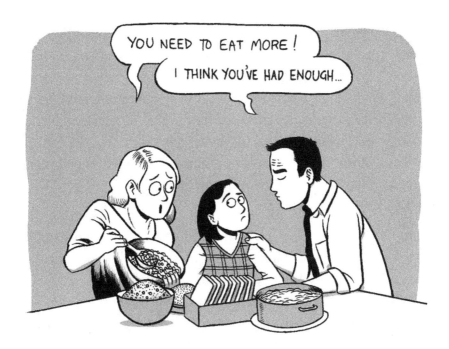

Parental unity is probably the most important skill required to manage your adolescent with anorexia. The best chance you have of defeating the illness is by presenting a united front against the anorexia. Decisions will need to be made jointly and you will both need to provide a consistent message regarding every aspect of refeeding, your expectations of your child and their behavior otherwise the anorexia will divide you both and ultimately defeat your efforts to get your child better.

Enhancing parental authority is critical and one of the strongest predictors of recovery. The FBT manual emphasizes that parents *"need to be on the same page, the same line, and the same letter."* A trial by Ellison et al showed that greater weight gain was achieved when the parents were united and were able to take control. [11]

WHY DO PARENTS STRUGGLE TO WORK TOGETHER?

Parents normally approach the parental role with very different views on parenting. This is due to an individual's personal experience of being parented. As we grow up in our families of origin we internalize a model of our own parents. This is called the internal working model of parenting. How many of us have said "When I am a parent, I will never do that to my children" and then one day when we are parents we suddenly realize that we are acting and doing exactly as our own parents did.

Having different views on parenting is not usually a major problem when a family is travelling along smoothly. Most families can accommodate the different values and expectations that each parent brings from their past. Sometimes one parent will take on the "soft" role and the other the "tougher" parent. Children quickly adapt to each parent's style and expectations. However, when you are dealing with an adolescent with anorexia any parental disunity becomes disastrous. Anorexia quickly splits the parents by hurling abuse at the stronger parent and trying to gain sympathy or an ally from the weaker parent resulting in parental disunity.

When dealing with an adolescent with anorexia, parenting all of a sudden becomes foreign and parents begin to doubt their own parenting abilities. They are shocked that their normal parental capacities and strategies no longer appear to work. The new family crisis results in instability and leaves parents at a loss to know what and how to manage their adolescent. Parental disunity and criticism immediately shows its ugly face when one parent tries to manage a situation and fails. This can result in the other parent becoming critical of their partner's efforts, feeling that they know a better way to manage the situation only to also fail. Unfortunately when this happens the anorexia is the only victor.

Contributing to parental disunity is the continual exposure to your child's distress. A distressed child raises parental anxiety and leaves parents feeling helpless. Your anorexic adolescent, when confronted with food will become very distressed, will most likely scream and cry, and will inevitably tug at your heart strings as you watch them suffer. When this happens it is normal for parents to become distressed and overwhelmed by a sense of helplessness and confusion and it may convince you to reduce their food. You need to become aware if your response to your child is driven by your own anxiety in response to their distress. You will need to forge through your own anxiety and stay on task in order to get your child better.

Parents need to realize that refeeding an anorexic adolescent IS NOT normal parenting. It is a prescription to get your child healthy and weight-restored, therefore as a prescription, it needs to be administered in exactly the same way by both parents.

A good way for parents to think about this statement is this: if a doctor gave your child a prescription to take one antibiotic tablet every four hours, that is probably how you would both administer the medication. Both parents would adhere to the prescription and dosage. It would be ridiculous to think that one parent would change the dose to 2 tablets four times a day or perhaps administer the medication in an ad hoc way. If you can think of "refeeding" as a prescription that you **BOTH** must adhere to and administer as per the prescription, it makes working together much easier as individual values will not interfere with the task.

YOUR EMOTIONAL RESPONSE TO YOUR CHILD

There are four emotional ways parents respond to their child – apathy, sympathy, empathy and compassion.

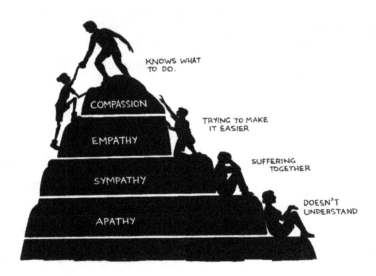

Apathy *Dave!*

At the bottom there is apathy. Apathy means that you are disconnected to what is happening. Parents usually respond this way when they struggle to understand anorexia and what's going on for their child. Apathy is evident when you hear parents say, "Why don't they just eat?" or "How hard can it be to eat, they are just stubborn." The message you give your child is "I don't understand what's happening to you. I am not connected to what you are feeling."

Sympathy *Me at mealtime when I don't directly instruct Grace to eat*

Parents usually have a lot of sympathy because they care for their child, and seeing them distressed usually results in too much sympathy. Sympathy actually means "suffering together." Too much sympathy won't get your child healthy. The message you give with sympathy is, "I feel so sorry for you, and I understand how hard it is for you that I just can't make it any harder for you so I am not going to insist that you eat everything you need to eat. I will just sit with you and share your suffering with you." If your only response is sympathy both you and your child will be stuck.

Empathy *Me when offering low calorie drinks*

Then we move to empathy. When parents are empathetic they can really understand how hard it is for their child. Your child also knows that you understand how hard it is for them, so you both stay connected with that shared understanding. Empathetic parents feel so connected with their child's distress that they just want to make eating as easy as possible for their child so they agree to feed them what makes them happy, which is usually light food or what your child calls "safe foods". Whilst you may see some improvement with lots of empathy, both you and your child are stuck. Again, with too much empathy your child will never attain full recovery. Full recovery means normalized, healthy eating and this will not occur if your child never becomes comfortable eating everything, including fear foods that they ate prior to the anorexia. When you are too empathetic the message you give your child is "I understand and will make this as easy as I can for you at the expense of full recovery."

Compassion *Where I strive to be all the time*

Finally there is compassion. When you are compassionate, you really understand your child's predicament. You really understand what your child is battling with, but you also understand that if you don't get your child out of this predicament they will never recover and lead a normal adolescent life. With compassion you are resolved to make things better for them no matter how hard it is. The message you give is, "I understand you, and I feel with you, but I am going to get you better. I am going to get you out of that place where you are so stuck."

Given the intensity of the treatment, you will swing between these four emotions but ultimately if you are to get your child better you will need to be functioning for most of the time (90-95%) with compassion.

Compassion is easy to give someone who wants it, but remember that part of your child doesn't want your help, they want to be thin and will fight to remain thin; therefore, you need to remain committed to your task in the face of your child's displays of anger towards you. Be prepared that your child will not give up without a fight and remember the saying "United we stand, divided we fall." Your child needs you both to be united.

A good way to stay on track is to develop mantras that can be repeated internally when you feel frustrated and/or feel like giving in to your child. Following are several examples:

— *My child needs me to get through this.*

— *We are going to get through this one meal, one day at a time.*

— *They are scared and can't make appropriate decisions.*

— *It's not my child saying that to me, it's the anorexia.*

— *They need to eat to get healthy. This is the only way to get my child back.*

— *They need us to help them. They can't fight anorexia on their own.*

— *Food is the only thing that will get rid of their distress.*

— *Their aggressive behavior is a cry for my help.*

— *Anorexia is tormenting them; all I have to do is feed them.*

It is important to remember not to become discouraged when things go wrong and inevitably there are times when, despite your best efforts, they will. This is a time when you should strengthen your resolve and plan how you will do things differently the next time. Below is a problem-solving wheel many parents find useful, and should be used frequently as it promotes support and communication between parents.

PROBLEM SOLVING WHEEL

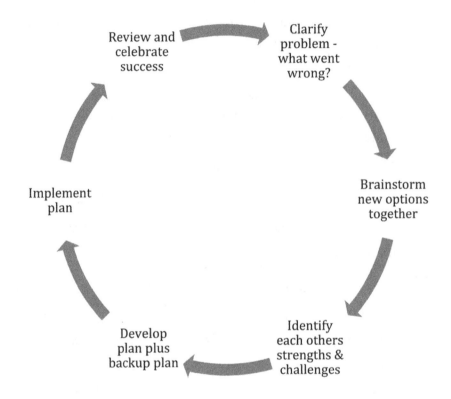

HOW SHOULD I RESPOND
TO MY CHILD?

WHAT MAKES CHILDREN AND ADOLESCENTS FEEL SAFE?

One of the primary tasks of parenting is to raise secure children. In order to do this parents need to provide a consistent and reliable environment where children feel safe to explore and push boundaries knowing that their parents are available should they sometimes fail. In order for this to occur, parents need to provide appropriate boundaries regarding what **is,** and what **is not,** acceptable behavior. This is called authoritative and nurturing parenting, where the child has trust and confidence in their parents. Nothing is more frightening to a child than feeling out of control compounded with the knowledge that their parents also feel out of control.

Anorexia makes your child feel totally out of control despite their illusion and protests that they are in control. If they were in control they would not compromise their health to the extent that they are. Unfortunately anorexia also makes parents feel out of control.

If parents show signs that they are intimidated either by the anorexia or by their child's behavior, the child will feel they cannot depend on their parent and that their parents have abandoned them when they need them most. Alternatively your display of being intimidated by the anorexia can also make your child feel they are all powerful and therefore they are the only ones that can keep themselves safe. If your child cannot depend on you to make them feel safe that only leaves the anorexia to depend on; therefore your child will continue to be ruled by their anorexia. This self-dependency and dependency on anorexia will also make your child resistant to seek help from others.

You need to respond to your child in a calm and non-critical manner despite your child's displays of distress and anger. You need to show your child that you are in control of the situation and that you know what you are doing despite the fact that internally you may be feeling equally distressed and unsure of what you are doing. Your firm belief that you are doing the right thing will emotionally contain and make your child safe. If parents - the people they have trusted all their life - can't help them, then they automatically think that no one can and therefore they are unsafe.

Practical exercise that demonstrates feeling contained – Close your eyes for a moment and picture you are in a room with a group of friends and there is a fire in the next room. A firefighter comes running into your room very anxious, stressed, waving their arms screaming and repeatedly yelling that there is a fire in the next room that is out of control. They state that they are unsure that they can put out the fire and also unsure if they can get everyone out quickly and safely. Despite the firefighter's best intentions, their lack of confidence immediately raises your anxiety and fear that you can die, that you cannot trust them to get you out safely. The firefighter's actions have also made you doubtful. You begin to question if you should listen to them and if they really know what they are doing.

Now picture the same scenario but this time the firefighter comes into your room very calmly stating that there is a fire in the next room and that everything is under control, the fire will be extinguished shortly, there is nothing to worry about and if you just follow their instructions and remain calm they will get everyone out safely. This firefighter will automatically make you feel contained and safe.

You need to respond to your child in a similar manner – as the calm and confident firefighter so your child can feel contained and safe in the belief that you will and can help them. *The message to your child is that you will keep them safe and will not let anything happen to them.*

When you are dealing with your child, if you feel that you are going to lose control and get angry, make an excuse and walk away and get your partner to take over. Getting angry with your child will only make them feel guilty. It also sends a message to the anorexia that it is wearing you down and winning; therefore, all the anorexia needs to do is to continue the behavior so as to frustrate you sufficiently to convince you to give up.

Sometimes parents become frightened or equally distressed by their child's displays of anger and distress, and they feel that by pushing food they are making their child more distressed. This is anorexia's way to keep you distracted from what you need to do. The only way to relieve your child's distress is to get your child back to a healthy weight, therefore you need to stay on task and feed your child. Your child may temporarily feel happy when you don't make them eat more, but internally they will continue to be tormented by their anorexia if they remain at an unhealthy weight with insufficient nutrition for their body to function and support their physical development.

HOW DO I MANAGE
MY CHILD'S DISTRESS?

Many parents struggle to understand and manage their child's distress. Watching your child feel out of control, crying, screaming, and extremely distressed makes parents feel very vulnerable, powerless, and just as distressed as their child.

Most children suffering with anorexia will become very distressed coping with the quantity of food they are required to eat and the consequent weight gain. Both food and weight gain usually make your child feel they are losing control. Some adolescents become so distressed that they may engage in self-harm, threats of suicide, attempts to run away and become abusive towards their parents. You need to remember why your child is so distressed (refer to the factors outlined on pages 21-27). Hopefully as your child becomes healthier these behaviors should diminish. Unfortunately for some adolescents the anorexic thoughts may take a little longer, and for some adolescents they may take 12-18 months to completely disappear. Keep in mind that your child has sustained a trauma to the brain, therefore the brain needs time to recover. Example, if your child had sustained a serious leg fracture it would take a considerable amount of time for your child to gain the full use of his/her leg and recommence competitive running.

Nancy Zucker eloquently describes emotions as being similar to waves. Nancy's analogy helps parents visually understand what is happening for their child when they become distressed. It also helps parents to become aware how their child's emotions escalate as they climb the "emotional wave."[12]

When your child is exposed to what they feel is an unmanageable situation it increases their emotional energy. The closer your child gets to the crest of their emotional wave the greater the intensity of their distress. Example, when your child is confronted with food, your child's distress (emotional energy) will start to rise. As your child climbs up the emotional wave your child's ability to think clearly and regain emotional control decreases. When your child has reached the crest of their emotional wave they will be in a state of extreme emotional arousal and at this point their fear and emotions are so intense that your child cannot respond to logic or reasoning. As your child climbs the wave every level usually requires a different response.

Your child needs your help to come down from their emotional wave and return to a calmer state. Your task is to learn how to calm your child and help them to learn skills so they can come down safely from their emotional wave.

When your child is climbing the wave, this is the time to intervene with distraction and self-soothing techniques. At this point your child has some ability to concentrate and possibly self-regulate. However, once on the crest of the wave, talking and logic no longer work, and it is best to provide some physical comfort for your child such as a hug and tell them you will keep them safe. It is best to intervene before your child reaches the crest.

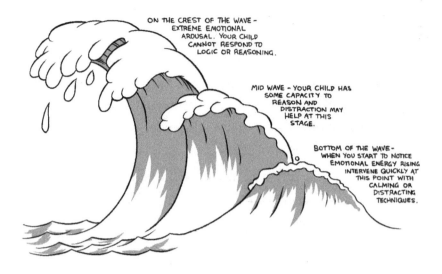

ON THE CREST OF THE WAVE –
EXTREME EMOTIONAL
AROUSAL. YOUR CHILD
CANNOT RESPOND TO
LOGIC OR REASONING.

MID WAVE – YOUR CHILD HAS
SOME CAPACITY TO
REASON AND
DISTRACTION MAY
HELP AT THIS
STAGE.

BOTTOM OF THE WAVE –
WHEN YOU START TO NOTICE
EMOTIONAL ENERGY RISING
INTERVENE QUICKLY AT
THIS POINT WITH
CALMING OR
DISTRACTING
TECHNIQUES.

HOW DO I GET MY CHILD DOWN FROM THE EMOTIONAL WAVE?

Distraction is the process of thinking about something so intently that you lose focus on the original thought/situation that created the distress. Distraction also temporarily takes your attention off strong emotions. Parents use distraction techniques when they know their child will face or is facing a distressing situation. For anorexic adolescents the most distressing situations usually involve food and eating either pre, post or during the actual meal time. Therefore the distraction strategy you decide upon should coincide with the time you feel your child's anxiety will be at its peak.

→ **Following a meal** – Anorexia can make your child feel extremely guilty after a meal as they may be flooded with self-loathing thoughts and thoughts of failure due to loss of control. It is usually when your child is in this state that they are tempted to purge the calories they have consumed either by vomiting and/or exercising. After meals is a good time to introduce activities that distract them from these thoughts.

→ **Prior to a meal** – Many adolescents become very agitated prior to eating as they think about the quantity and foods their parents will make them eat. They will feel they need to know what their parents are making and what they are putting in the meal. It is easier to keep your child out of the kitchen and probably a good time to use soothing techniques and/or distraction techniques.

→ **During the meal** – Eating the meal can also be a difficult time so this is when you would use distraction. Many families sit together during meals and try and initiate conversations about daily events unrelated to food that will distract their child; many will allow their adolescent to watch their favorite TV shows, YouTube videos, or play games whilst eating as a distraction.

It is up to you to know your enemy – the anorexia. You need to know when the anorexia is at its strongest. Is it the morning meal or evening meal? When the anorexia is at its strongest, be more prepared with strategies and a plan to manage your child's distress. Lunch

Your child's distress is not just restricted to food, eating, and weight gain as there will be occasions throughout the treatment when your child will become distressed in response to thoughts about their body image especially when clothes become tighter and/or they see their reflection in the mirror. Learn to read those situations quickly before your child climbs too high on their emotional wave. Remember the lower on the wave they are, the easier it is to get them back down on the beach.

Parents usually know their child's likes and dislikes so any distraction strategy you use will usually be more successful if it is centered around your child's interests.

Following are strategies that many parents have found useful. You can be creative and come up with your own as no one knows your child better than you. Remember the strategy needs to help your child fully focus their attention on the activity you present. Early on in treatment the strategy cannot involve a large expenditure of calories; therefore strategies need to be sedentary. As your child gains more weight, activities can be more active like going for a short walk etc. However, you need to be guided by your FBT therapist regarding any additional exercise.

Tummy?

DISTRACTION STRATEGIES

→ ZENTANGLE – Is an intricate art form that requires a lot of concentration and many artistic adolescents usually love this technique. It is normally called "yoga for the mind."

→ COLORING-IN BOOKS are usually very relaxing and mind consuming.

→ TV and YouTube are great distractions especially 'Funniest Home Videos' and 'Funniest Cat/Animal Videos'. Cat videos are actually the most watched Youtube videos and very funny and distractive.

→ CREATIVE ARTS – If your child is creative and loves making things, then be creative with them.

→ AUDIO BOOKS – If your child was an avid reader, listening to one of their favorite novels whilst eating can take their mind off the meal.

→ ONLINE FREE GAMES - jigsaw puzzles, games etc.

SELF-SOOTHING STRATEGIES

→ Listening to relaxing meditation/zen music. The PANDORA app has a wide range of relaxing music you can download free.

→ Breathing and Calming Apps – 'Smiling Mind'; 'Fast Calm'

→ Guided meditations and visualization – There are many apps or you can guide your child.

Remember the distraction needs to be interesting,
absorbing, immersive and easy to focus for
a sustained period.

Parent Reflection on
Distraction Techniques During ReFeeding

Our FBT therapist introduced our daughter to "Zentangle" or "yoga for the mind." During mealtimes our daughter would create her own Zentangle pictures, which helped her through many tough meals. They were creative, required attention to detail and, more importantly, calmed her. The drawings were beautiful and she was proud of her artwork.

Our daughter also discovered a breathing method to calm her mind during particularly distressing mealtimes. She would imagine a "square" and, beginning at the bottom of the square, breathe in for four counts up to the top of the square, hold her breath for four counts across the top of the square, breathe out for four counts from the top to the bottom of the square, then hold her breath for four counts for the final bottom "right to left" count. This would slow down her heart rate and somewhat help to relieve her anxiety.

Following mealtimes, we discovered that it was important to distract our daughter from her distress. Often we would go for a 20-minute walk together. This would give our daughter the opportunity to talk. Or not! Either way, silent or conversational, she generally felt more relaxed and grounded after a walk.

Alternatively, after meals we would play table tennis! We did not own a table tennis table so we did the next best thing and bought bats, balls and a portable net, which clamped onto our dining room table. We played hours of table tennis as a family and we all became extremely competitive!

In addition, we invested in every season of "Friends" on DVD and our daughter watched two to three episodes per night after evening meals. She looked forward to this and it was wonderful to see her laugh again.

During the early days of refeeding we decided it was time to get a puppy, not only for our daughter but also for our whole family. Our younger children were deeply affected by the emotional rollercoaster of refeeding and our gorgeous dog gave - and continues to give - our daughter and her siblings so much love and comfort. Our daughter often says she just doesn't know what she would have done without our family dog. The puppy did not join us for mealtimes!

Anorexia Nervosa is a complex illness and we often felt we were learning "on the job." Every spare moment we had, we researched eating disorders through books, attending EDV meetings and seeking answers online via 'F.E.A.S.T. Around the Dinner Table Forum.' We also attended an eating disorder conference, which was enlightening, informative and gave us the opportunity to connect with other families of sufferers. We knew it was essential to gain as much information and knowledge as we could in order to help our daughter recover from her illness.

Written by a mother of a child, age 14, with Anorexia

SIMPLE TIPS TO HELP YOUR CHILD MANAGE THEIR ANXIETY

Current research shows that there is a major association between anxiety and eating disorders. A high percentage of adolescents with anorexia suffer from childhood anxiety; this is predictive of more severe ED symptoms.[13] It is expected that adolescents with premorbid anxiety will continue to be highly anxious following weight restoration. During anorexia your child will develop many unrealistic fears and thoughts about food that will exacerbate any pre-existing anxiety. Your child will also be affected with 'anticipatory anxiety', which means they will become very anxious thinking about confronting the next meal you are preparing even before you have presented the meal.

Put simply, anxiety is a result of thoughts convincing you that you will not cope with a certain situation or event. Example: *Thought* – I will not do any good on my exam. You keep worrying and ruminating on that thought continually until you convince yourself that you will fail despite all your efforts to study for the exam. You actually build a mental picture of yourself failing. By constantly thinking about the negative thought/outcome you continually **"reinforce"** it, and by reinforcing it you strengthen a negative neural pathway.

A good way to manage this anxiety is to replace the negative picture/thought with positive affirmations and creating a positive picture of getting an "A" for the exam. You need to repeat the positive affirmations, thoughts and visualize your success as often as you can throughout the day when you are calm. You will eventually convince your brain that you will get an "A." You are actually reprogramming your brain by creating new pathways and getting rid of the negative (anxiety) pathways and reducing anxiety.

THE NECESSITY OF EXPOSURE

An adolescent with anorexia and high levels of anxiety will usually develop thoughts and fears about certain foods that they have classed as "bad" together with the worrying consequences these foods will have on their body. The adolescent may also develop anxiety about eating in front of others or going out to eat in public. Their constant worrying about these issues will only reinforce the beliefs. Despite your child's anxiety you will need to help your child confront these fears by exposing them to what they fear. This is called **exposure therapy**. Therefore you will need to gently get your child to eat the feared foods and eat in public and with others. If you do not expose your child to what makes them anxious, full recovery is never achieved.

Many of these situations will induce anticipatory anxiety. A good way to help your child manage these situations and their anxiety is to teach your child deep-breathing exercises. A good strategy is to develop "check-in" points throughout the day. This is done by asking your child to sit comfortably, place their hands on their tummy, close their eyes, and take slow deep breaths to the bottom of their stomach and feel the rise and fall of their tummy as they concentrate on their breathing. You also ask them to visualize themselves being calm and present. They will need to do this for two minutes 10-12 times per day. Check-ins can also be helpful pre and post meals. This exercise can be done together or you can guide your child through the exercise. The constant repetition of check-ins aims to teach your child to self-regulate. Many parents also find the exercise useful in reducing their own stress and anxiety regarding refeeding.

RESOURCES
FOR PARENTS

BOOKS:

Anorexia and Other Eating Disorders - How to Help Your Child Eat Well and Be Well – Eva Musby

Help Your Teenager Beat an Eating Disorder – James Lock and Daniel LeGrange

Brave Girl Eating – Harriet Brown

Decoding Anorexia – Carrie Arnold

My Kid is Back – June Alexander & Daniel le Grange

Skills Based Learning for Caring for a Loved One with an Eating Disorder – Janet Treasure

Eating with your Anorexic: A Mother's Memoir – Laura Collins

Throwing Starfish across the Sea – C Bevan & L Collins

All books are available at https://www.bookdepository.com/ with free shipping.

WEBSITES:

www.maudsleyparents.org
Website explaining Family Based Treatment (FBT).

http://evamusby.co.uk/anorexia-help-your-child-eat-with-trust-not-logic/ &

http://evamusby.co.uk/videos-eating-disorder-anxiety-child/
Practice short videos for parents for meal support and how to engage in the eating disorder debate.

www.feast-ed.org
International organization for caregivers of eating disorder patients. Serves families by providing information and mutual support.

www.aroundthedinnertable.org
Forum with parents of children with eating disorders sharing strategies and stories.

http://www.eatingdisorders.org.au/
Eating Disorders Victoria. Eating Disorders Victoria (EDV) provides a comprehensive support and information service on all aspects of eating disorders.

www.ceed.org.au
Provides information and advice for carers.

www.mindfulnessforteens.com
Mindfulness resources for young people.

https://www.youtube.com/watch?v=G0T_2NNoC68
Hand Brain Model (Daniel Siegel)
What is happening to the brain when a child is distressed?

https://www.youtube.com/watch?v=wRKV1ltiSFc
Eating Disorders and neuroscience.

https://www.youtube.com/watch?v=W1YjNlF-U7M
What are Eating Disorders? by Brian Lask.

APPS:

<u>Smiling Mind</u>

<u>Fast Calm</u>

REFERENCES

1. Lock J & LeGrange D., *Treatment Manual for Anorexia Nervosa - A Family Based Approach,* Second Ed. 2013, Guilford Press, NY, London.

2. Doyle P, LeGrange D, Loeb K, Doyle A, Crosby R, Early response to Family-Based Treatment for adolescent Anorexia Nervosa, (2009), *Int J Eating Disorders,* 43(7):659-62

3. Lock J, Agras WS, Bryson S, Kraemer HC, (2005): Comparison of short and long-term family therapy for adolescent anorexia nervosa, *J AM Acad Child & Adolescent Psychiatry,* 44:632-639

4. Lock J, (2015): An Update on Evidence-Based Psychosocial Treatments for Eating Disorders in Children and Adolescents, *Journal of Clinical Child & Adolescent Psychology,* DOI: 10.1080/15374416.2014.971458

5. Lask B, & Frampton I, *Eating Disorders & the Brain,* 2011, Pub Wiley-Blackwell.

6. Nunn K, Hanstock T, & Lask B, *The Who's Who of the Brain,* 2008, Jessica Kingsley Pub. London & Philadelphia

7. Nunn K, Frampton I, Gordon I, Lask B, 2008: The Fault is not in her parents but in her insula – a neurobiological hypothesis of anorexia. *Eur Eat Disord Rev,* 16(5):355-60.

8. Kleiman S, Carroll I, Tarantino L, Bulik C, 2015: Gut Feelings: A role for the intestinal microbiota in anorexia nervosa? *Int J Eating Disorders,* 48:449-451

9. White H, Haycraft E, Madden S, Rhodes P, Miskovic-Wheatley J, Wallis A, Kohn M, Meyer C, 2014: How do parents of adolescent patients with anorexia nervosa interact with their child at mealtimes? *Int J Eating Disorders,* 48(1):72-80

10. Schebendach JE, Mayer LE, Devlin MJ, Attia E, Contento IR, Wolf RL, Walsh T., 2011, Food choice and diet variety in weight-restored patients with anorexia nervosa. *J Am Diet Assoc.* 111:732-736

11. Ellison R, Rhodes P, Madden S, Miskovic J, Wallis A, Billie A, Kohn M, Touyz S, 2012: Do the components of manualised family-based treatment for anorexia nervosa predict weight gain? *Int J Eating Disorders,* 45:609-614

12. Zucker N, 2008, Off the Cuff - A Parent Skills Book for the Management of Disordered Eating. Duke University Medical Centre.

13. Kaye W, Wierenga CE, Bailer UF, Simmons AN, Bischoff-Grethe A. 2013, Nothing Tastes as Good as Skinny Feels: The Neurobiology of Anorexia Nervosa. *Trends in Neuroscience,* 36(2).

* Estimates of prevalence of Anorexia obtained from the Eating Disorders Victoria website (http://www.eatingdisorders.org.au)

CPSIA information can be obtained
at www.ICGtesting.com
Printed in the USA
BVHW041925030820
585373BV00013B/333